Preface:

This is my low carb recipe book based on the recipes that I used to not only lose weight but become a healthier me. I have lost 75 lbs!! But it took years of many diets after diets, to realize that it has to be a life change and not just a diet to not only stop the 'yo-yo' of my weight, but become healthier and feel like a new person. ☺

Why Low Carb?

Carbs are usually the hardest to reduce from most people's diet. Carbs are the body's preferred energy source, just as gas fuels a car, carbs fuel your body. The problem is that too many of us indulge into baskets of bread, mashed potatoes, pasta, cake, and cupcakes laden with sugar. These types of carbs can get us into trouble. We all need some carbs in our diets, but they not created equal.

Refined carbohydrates like sugar and white bread raise blood sugar and offer little nutrition beyond calories. However more complex carbs such as whole grains, whole fruit, and vegetables are easier on blood sugar and are packed with valuable nutrients. In my recipes, I use more complex carbs such as fiber, fresh fruits, and non-starch veggies.

Using complex carbs will help you with weight loss, along with an exercise plan. Taking out those sugar laden carbs you will be so surprised at how much better you will feel!!!! ☺

Every recipe in this book has been carefully considered at how delicious, healthy & easy to prepare and cook. I often spend hours comparing ingredient choices before selecting for a recipe. Some recipes have created through much trial and error on taste vs healthy.

Most choices are common like reduced sodium chicken broth, light soy sauce, cheeses, and choice of meats and fresh veggies. There are a few items like Oat fiber and Phylum husks that are not as common, but these are carefully considered. These items are high in fiber, has no calories, and does not raise blood sugar, has a large range of health benefits such as risk from breast cancer, colon cancers, heart disease, and obesity (per research on MyPlate.gov).

A higher fiber diet can speed up weight loss and keep you feeling full.

**Note: I usually prepare snacks, muffins, and no carb bread ahead of time so I can have them on hand for easy access. Having these prepared ahead of time will make grabbing a quick snack easier and healthier. ☺

Index

SNACKS
Snack Stacks
Spinach Chips
Cheese Chips
Mozzarella Sticks
Creamy Shrimp Tacos

BREAKFAST
Mexican Scrambled Eggs
No Bread Breakfast Sandwich
Cauliflower Hash
No Carb Pancakes/Waffles
Classic Eggs and Bacon
Frittata Muffins
No Carb Bread

LUNCH, DINNER, SUPPER
Skillet Pork & Peppers
Stir-Fry Lemon and Garlic Chicken/Green Beans
Spinach Quiche
Zesty Grilled Hamburgers
Chicken & Broccoli Casserole
Cabbage Soup
Grilled Salmon w/Orange Sauce
Baked Tilapia
Kimmie's Tomato Soup
Low Carb Pizza Crust
Chicken & "Potato" Soup
Spinach Stuffed Chicken Breast

DESSERTS
Kimmie's Coconut Choc Chip Cookies
Salty Choc Treats
Ice Cream
Orange Cranberry Muffins
Coconut Cream with Berries
Kimmie's Chocolate Frosted Cookies

LOW CARB SMOOTHIES

SNACKS

Snacking is an effective way to fit extra nutrients into your diet and prevent overeating at mealtimes. According to a study published in "The Journal of Nutrition" in February 2010, approximately 97 percent of Americans snack, getting an average of 24 percent of their calories from snacks. With snacking providing this much of the day's calories, choosing healthy options is crucial.

Stack Snack

1 c. Cubed ham
6 Pickles cut into cubes
4 cheese sticks cut into cubes Toothpicks

1. Cut each item into the same size cubes.
2. Take 1 piece of each item and skewer with toothpick.

- You can use any type of cheese sticks. I prefer the Colby & Monterey Jack cheese sticks.

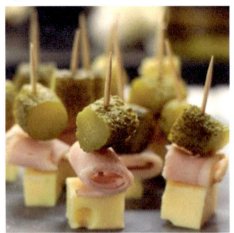

These stack snacks have always been my kids favorite snack because they had fun helping me make them. Not only are they no carb, but are a great tasting snack because the flavor combination on these skewers mimics that of a Cuban sandwich -- minus the bread. ☺

Spinach Chips

1 c. Baby spinach
¼ c. Parmesan cheese
Dash of cayenne pepper
2 tbls olive oil or coconut oil

Preheat oven to 350

1. Mix all ingredients together in a bowl making sure it is evenly coated.
2. Place on a greased baking sheet spacing each piece 1 inch a part
3. Bake for 8-10 minutes. Spinach should be crisp.

- You can add other flavoring like garlic or Italian seasonings.

Spinach is low in fat and even lower in cholesterol, spinach is high in niacin and zinc, as well as protein, fiber, vitamins A, C, E and K, thiamin, vitamin B6, folate, calcium, iron, magnesium, phosphorus, potassium, copper, and manganese. In other word, it's loaded with good things for every part of your body!

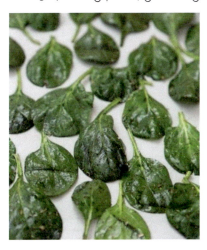

Cheese Chips

2 c. Colby/Monterey jack shredded cheese Pepperoni (optional)
Jalapeno peppers (optional)

Preheat oven to 425
1. Line baking sheet with foil and spray with non-sticking spray.
2. Place 1 large pinch of cheese & pat to spread into a "cookie" format.
3. Place about 2 inches apart (add optional toppings)
4. Bake for 6-8 minutes until browning on edges.

Chips should be crisp and ready to dip in salsa, alone, or with chosen toppings.

These chips are so easy to make and you can choose so many different toppings like pepperoni or jalapenos.

Mozzarella Sticks

8 mozzarella string cheese sticks
2 tbls parmesan cheese
1 large egg
1 tsp dried parsley
½ tsp garlic salt
¼ tsp dried oregano

Preheat oven to 400

1. Cut the mozzarella sticks in half crosswise (you should have 16 short sticks)
2. Place the parmesan cheese, parsley, garlic salt & oregano in a small bowl.
3. **Place the beaten egg in a small bowl**
4. Roll the sticks in the parmesan cheese, and then the egg. Drip off excess.
5. Place on greased baking sheet and freeze for 1 hour.
6. Take from freezer and bake for 10-13 minutes until golden brown.

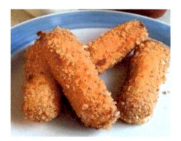

Creamy Shrimp Tacos

Taco shells

½ lb 225 g shredded cheese

½ teaspoon ground cumin

Taco shells

1. Preheat the oven to 400°F. Mix cheese and cumin. Form six or eight piles on a baking sheet lined with parchment paper. Leave plenty of room in between piles, or the cheese might melt together.
2. Bake in the oven for 10-15 minutes or until the cheese is bubbling with golden brown patches – burned cheese doesn't taste good. Let cool for 30 seconds.
3. Place a rack over the sink.
4. Carefully, place the cheese platelets on the rack.
5. Let cool and serve with a filling of your choice.

Creamy shrimp filling

1. Sauté the shrimps in a hot pan with coconut oil, garlic and chili until the the shrimp have turned a nice pink color.
2. Salt to taste. Set aside and let cool.
3. Mix all other ingredients and add fried shrimps. Mix well and apply to the taco shells.
4. Salt and pepper to taste. Serve immediately!.

Creamy shrimp filling ⅔ lb 300 g 2 tablespoons coconut oil 1 1 cup 2⅖ dl _mayonnaise_ ¼ cup 60 ml fresh cilantro, chopped salt and pepper

List of my quick grab snacks

Almonds
Grapes
Blackberries
Strawberries
Blueberries
Cheese cubes
Apples
Slim jims Pickles
Cucumbers
Hard boiled eggs
Celery
Ham cubes
Sugar-free jello
Deviled eggs
Tuna fresh from can
Pork Rinds
Stacks*
My low carb fruit smoothies' ☺

Snacking helps keep you from getting overly hungry in between meals and then overeating at your next meal. So next time you start to feel hungry a couple hours before lunch or dinner, don't try to wait until the meal. Instead, eat a small healthy snack to tide you over. Combine a carbohydrate-rich food like whole grains, fruits or vegetables with protein foods like nuts or dairy products for the most filling snacks

Breakfast

Why is eating breakfast important? Many studies, in both adults and children, have shown that breakfast eaters tend to weigh less than breakfast skippers.

Why? One theory suggests that eating a healthy breakfast can reduce hunger throughout the day, and help people make better food choices at other meals. While it might seem you could save calories by skipping breakfast, this is not an effective strategy. Typically, hunger gets the best of breakfast-skippers, and they eat more at lunch and throughout the day.

Another theory behind the breakfast-weight control link implies that eating breakfast is part of a healthy lifestyle that includes making wise food choices and balancing calories with exercise.

It's worth noting that most studies linking breakfast to weight control loss looked at a healthy breakfast containing protein and/or whole grains -- not meals loaded with fat and calories.

The following breakfast recipes are just a few that you can do, I just wanted to create some breakfast choices that are different because eating just scrambled eggs every day got old.

However, eating scrambled eggs and turkey bacon is a great choice. ☺

Mexican Scrambled Eggs

Do you want more inspiration for your low-carb breakfast? Here's a great spicy start of the day! A wonderful mix of creamy scrambled eggs and a fresh taste of spicy jalapeños.

6 eggs
1 – 2 scallions
15 – 20 pickled jalapeños, finely chopped
1 tomato finely chopped
4 oz. 100 g shredded cheese
2 tablespoons butter, for frying Salt and pepper

1. Finely chop the spring onions, jalapeños and tomatoes. Fry in butter for 3 minutes on medium heat.
2. Beat the eggs and pour into the pan and scramble for 2 minutes before adding cheese and seasoning.

Serving suggestion: Avocados, lettuce and dressing.

No Bread Breakfast Sandwich

Looking for a great low-carb breakfast? How about hot sandwiches without bread? You can do eggs over easy and a delicious filling of cheese and ham or any other of your favorites.

2 tablespoons butter
1 oz. 30 g ham
2 oz. 60 g cheddar cheese or provolone cheese or Edam cheese, cut in thick slices
Salt and pepper
A few drops of tabasco or Worcestershire sauce

1. Fry the eggs over easy (on both sides) on medium heat. Salt and pepper to taste.
2. Place the ham/pastrami/cold cuts on two eggs, then cheese and an egg on top.
3. Sprinkle a few drops of Tabasco or Worcestershire sauce if you want, and serve immediately.

Cauliflower Hash

1 c. chopped cauliflower
1 c. Sausage
¼ onion
¼ bellpepper
1 tsp Olive oil
Salt & pepper to taste

1. Cook sausage in a skillet until brown. Drain any grease.
2. Add cauliflower, seasoning, onion, & bell pepper.
3. Cook on low heat for 15 minutes until cauliflower is tender.

- I also will use link sausage (chopped).
- You can use other veggies too☺

The cauliflower takes the place of rice. Cauliflower does have carbs however they are the 'good' carbs. Cauliflower has great benefits too, for instance, one serving of cauliflower contains 77 percent of the recommended daily value of vitamin C. It's also a good source of vitamin K, protein, thiamin, riboflavin, niacin, magnesium, phosphorus, fiber, vitamin B6, folate, pantothenic acid, potassium, and manganese.

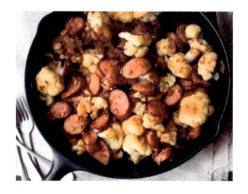

No Carb Pancakes/Waffles

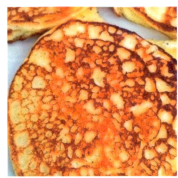

2 eggs
1 c. Oat Fiber (optional)
2 oz cream cheese
2 tsp cinnamon
1 pinch of salt
2 tsp Truvia sweetener

1. Mix all ingredients together on medium speed in a mixer. Blending well.
2. Heat skillet (or waffle maker) on medium heat
3. Pour 1/3 c. batter into pan (or into waffle maker)
4. When edges brown flip. When both sides are light brown remove from pan.
5. Eat with Sukrin syrup* (pic on last page)

Classic Eggs and Bacon

A classic low-carb breakfast that never gets old. Here with fried cherry tomatoes, herbs and spices. Eat as many eggs as you need to feel satisfied. Choose your bacon carefully, preferably organic and with as few additives as possible.

Eggs
Bacon
Tomatoes (optional)
Parsley

1. Fry the bacon in a pan until crispy and put aside on a plate.
2. Fry the eggs in the bacon grease any way you like them. Cut the cherry tomatoes in half and fry them at the same time.
3. Season with salt and pepper.

Frittata Muffins

½ c shredded Colby-Monterey jack cheese
3 eggs – beaten
1 c. onions & pepper chopped
1 tsp baking soda
½ c Oat Fiber*
Salt/pepper to taste

Preheat oven to 425

1. Mix all ingredients together making sure of no lumps
2. Spray muffin pan with cooking spray
3. Pour mixture into pan
4. Bake for 11-13 min (fork or toothpick should come out clean)

*Note : You don't have to use the oat fiber. It does make the consistency for cake like. ☺

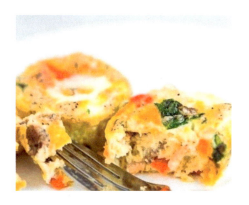

NO Carb Bread

3 eggs (separate)
2 oz cream cheese
¼ tsp cream of tartar
¼ tsp baking powder ½ c Oat Fiber* Pinch
of salt

Preheat oven to 425

1. Mix the egg yolks, cream cheese, cream of tartar, baking powder, Oat fiber in a mixer and blend well until smooth
2. Set aside
3. Next mix the eggs whites and salt and mix on high speed until the mixture is stiff.
4. Take the egg yolk mixture and fold gently in to the egg white mixture.
5. Place by the spoonful on to a greased baking sheet
6. Bake for 11-13 minutes or until golden brown

Note: You can use these for toast, to make a sandwich, or use as hamburger buns. ☺ Also note that for the best 'fluffy' bread advice is that as soon as you fold the mixtures together, to put them right into the oven. Do not let the mixture sit.

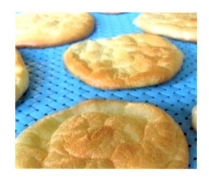

Lunch, Dinner, Supper

Note *** There are many variations that you can do to these recipes, but these are my favorites. ☺

Skillet Pork & Peppers

Salt/pepper
2 tsp dried oregano
1 tsp garlic powder
1 tsp smoked paprika
1 lb of cubed pork
1 tbsp olive oil
1 medium onion – chopped
1 medium bell pepper
1 tsp rosemary (dried)
2 tbls water

1. Take the first four ingredients in a large bowl, place the cubed pork and toss until evenly coated
2. Heat 2 tsp of oil in a large sauté pan over med/high heat.
3. Add pork mixture to skillet and sear for 2 min on each side, transfer to plate and set aside
4. Add remaining tsp of oil to pan, reduce heat to medium.
5. Add onion, garlic, rosemary, peppers, and water and cook until they are tender
6. Return Pork to the pan, reduce heat to low and cook for 5 min

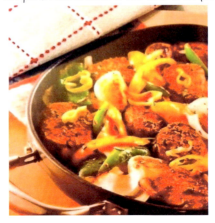

Stir Fry Lemon & Garlic Chicken & Green beans

1 tsp soy sauce
1 ½ lbs of boneless/skinless chicken diced into bite size cubes
1 tbsp olive oil
2 C. Green beans (I use fresh)
½ tsp diced garlic
¼ c lemon juice – freshly squeezed
Sesame seeds (optional)

1. In a large sauce pan, heat olive oil.
2. Add chicken and sauté until cooked
3. Add green beans, garlic, sesame seeds and lemon juice
4. Cook for 8-10 min until green beans are tender

*Note: You can substitute asparagus for green beans

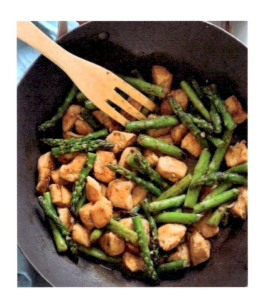

Spinach Quiche

1 c shredded cheese
4 eggs – 1 beaten, 3 for quiche
1/3 c minced onion
1 tsp Italian seasoning
1 c baby spinach- chopped
1 c low fat milk
1 ½ c shredded cheese for crust
2 tbsp cream cheese
¾ Oat Fiber *

Preheat oven to 425

1. Place Mozzarella cheese & cream cheese in a microwave safe bowl for 1 min Stir and replace in microwave for 30 sec
2. Wet hands and roll into ball then place on pizza stone or greased baking sheet.
3. Poke holes with fork to prevent bubbling
4. Bake for 8-10 min or until golden brown
5. Take crust and place in a pie pan or casserole dish
6. In a large bowl mix the 3 eggs, Italian seasonings, salt/pepper, onion, milk and remaining shredded cheese
7. Pour mixture in top of crust and bake for 30-35 min until the center is firm to touch.

*Note: Oat Fiber is optional ☺

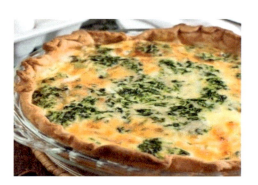

Low Carb Burritos

Low carb Tortillas (see pics)
1 lb of ground beef
1 packet of taco seasoning (I use low sodium)
1 c shredded cheese
Salt/pepper to taste
Salsa

Preheat oven to 350

1. Bake tortillas for 5-8 min until golden brown, set aside.
2. Cook ground beef, drain grease
3. Place the tortillas onto a plate and add your favorite toppings to tortillas and roll.
4. Top with cheese and return to oven until is melted.

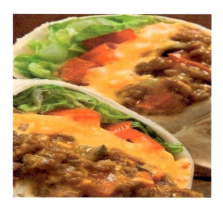

Zesty Grilled Hamburgers

1 lb of ground beef
1 tsp Worcestershire sauce
1 tsp mince onion (dried)
1 tsp A1
½ tsp cayenne pepper Salt/pepper to taste

1. In a large bowl combine all ingredients together
2. Take and roll handful into a ball and flatten into patties
3. Grill until desired temperature (well-done, med well, etc)

*Note eat hamburgers with my low carb bread or wrapped in lettuce ☺

Chicken & Broccoli "Casserole"

4 chicken breasts
1 can cream of chicken soup
2 c. shredded cheese
1 box frozen broccoli spears
1 bag of chopped cauliflower*
Chicken bouillon cube
½ onion

Preheat oven to 350

1. Boil chicken in bouillon cube and onion until chicken is cooked.
2. Remove, let cool, then cut into 2 inch cubes
3. Cool the broccoli in the broth until tender.
4. Remove and place broccoli, cauliflower, and chicken in a casserole dish.
5. Stir in 1 c of the shredded cheese, then place the remaining cheese on top of the mixture.
6. Bake for 15 min until cheese is bubbly.

*Note : The cauliflower is in the place of rice ☺

Cabbage Soup

½ head of cabbage – chopped
1 carton low sodium chicken broth
½ can diced tomatoes
Salt/pepper to taste

1. Place ingredients in a 4 ½ quart pan.
2. Cook for 20 min on medium heat.

Note***   Cabbage, which is often lumped into the same category as lettuce because of their similar appearance, is actually a part of the cruciferous vegetable family.

Cruciferous vegetables like cabbage, kale, and broccoli are notorious for being chock-full of beneficial nutrients. If you are trying to improve your diet, cruciferous vegetables should be at the very top of your grocery list.

Cabbage can vary in color from green to red and purple, and the leaves can be smooth or crinkled. With less than 20 calories per half cup cooked, it is a vegetable worth making room on your plate for. Choose a cabbage that is heavy for its size. Make sure the leaves are tight and firm as loose leaves indicate an older cabbage. Store cabbage in the refrigerator for up to two weeks. Cabbage can be eaten raw, steamed, boiled, roasted, sautéed, or stuffed. The sulfurous odor often associated with cabbage only develops when the cabbage is overcooked. The longer a cabbage is cooked, the stronger the odor becomes.   Quick tips for eating more cabbage: ☐Keep it simple and drizzle roasted chopped cabbage with olive oil, cracked black pepper, and minced garlic ☐Add shredded cabbage to a fresh green salad.

Grilled Salmon with Orange Sauce

1 orange – squeeze juice and zest
1 tbls rice vinegar
½ c of sukrin brown sugar
4 tsp soy sauce
Cayenne pepper to taste (optional)*
2-4 salmon fillets

1. Combine first 5 ingredients in a small sauce pan and bring to boil.
2. Reduce heat and simmer for 3 min
3. Remove from heat and set aside
4. Grill salmon over high heat, cooking each side approximately 5 min or until fish flakes apart easily.
5. Place salmon on plates and spoon the sauce over your fillets

*Note: you can also use 1 tsp of canned chipotle pepper in adobe sauce instead of cayenne pepper.

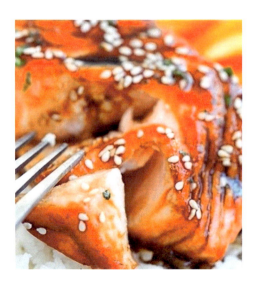

Baked Tilapia

2 Tilapia fillets
2 tsp of olive oil
1 lemon, sliced
1 c. Rotel
2 sheets of aluminum foil

Preheat oven to 425

1. Place 1 fillet in each sheet of foil
2. Put ½ c of Rotel onto each filler
3. Place ½ the lemon onto each fillet
4. Drizzle with olive oil
5. Wrap foil tightly
6. Bake for 25 min

Serve with broccoli or your favorite veggie ☺

Note**** Facts about Tilapia : One of the most important aspects of tilapia is its impressive protein content, making up more than 15% of our daily requirement in a single serving. Protein is an essential part of our diet, particularly animal proteins, because they can be enzymatically broken down into composite amino acids and reassembled into usable proteins in the human body. Protein is directly linked to proper growth and development of organs, membranes, cells, and muscles. It is particularly important that children consume adequate amounts of protein to ensure that they develop properly. They also are necessary for muscle growth, cellular repair, and proper metabolic activity of numerous organ systems.

Weight Loss: Unlike many other animal products, fish like tilapia are high in protein but low in calories and fats. This can be a good way to reduce your caloric intake, while still giving your body all of the necessary nutrients it needs to function properly. Fish is often turned to as a dietary option for people trying to lose weight, without starving themselves with crash diets.

Kimmie's Tomato Soup

1 Can of Tomato sauce
1 tbls of Basil
1 tbls of Red pepper flakes
1 tbls of minced garlic
4 oz of cream cheese
1 tbls of olive oil

1. Take the olive oil, basil, red pepper flakes and garlic in a sauce pan and brown the garlic.
2. Transfer to a medium pot and add the tomato sauce and cream cheese.
3. Simmer on low for 10 minutes

Note: you can add more or less of the basil and red pepper flakes.

Low Carb Pizza Crust

1 ½ C. shredded mozzarella cheese
¾ C Oat Fiber (optional)
2 tbsp cream cheese
1 egg, beaten
Garlic powder to taste
Pepperoni
Pizza sauce
Your favorite toppings

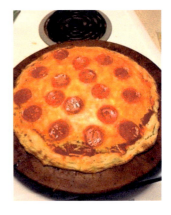

Preheat oven to 425

1. Put mozzarella & cream cheese in a microwave bowl & microwave for 1 min. Stir & replace in microwave for 30 sec
2. Stir in beaten egg & oat fiber
3. Wet hands & roll dough in to a ball and spread on a pizza stone or greased baking sheet. Poke holes in the dough with a fork to prevent bubbling.
4. Sprinkle with garlic powder (optional, your choice)
5. Put in oven for 8-10 min until golden brown
6. Top with your favorite toppings, then cook for 8-10 until cheese browns.

Note* Also this crust can be used for pizza sticks!!! Or just a cheese pizza ☺

Chicken & "Potato" Soup

1 Carton Low sodium chicken broth
1 c. chopped cauliflower
¼ c. onion
¼ c. celery
1 c. half & half cream
1 large chicken breast Salt & pepper to taste

1. Cook chicken in broth until chicken is done. (about 10 min)
2. Remove, cool, then cut into cubes.
3. Add Cauliflower, onion, celery, half & Half cream, cubed chicken
4. Cook for 15 min, Soup should have a nice creamy broth.
5. If you want a thicker broth, you can add cream of tartar (½ tsp) Enjoy!!

Spinach Stuffed Chicken Breast

4 large chicken breasts (pound flat)
1 c. spinach (chopped)
1 tsp minced garlic
¼ c parmesan cheese Toothpicks

Preheat oven 425

1. Mix cheese, spinach, garlic, & parmesan cheese.
2. Place a large spoonful onto each pounded chicken breast.
3. Spread evenly, then roll the beast and place a toothpick to hold
4. Cook for 20 min or until chicken is golden brown.

- Serve with your favorite green veggie ☺

Kimmie's Homemade Chicken Soup

1 Carton of low sodium Chicken broth
½ can diced tomatoes
1 c. Spinach (chopped)
1 large chicken breast cut into squares Salt & Pepper to taste

1. Boil chicken in broth, until chicken is cooked (about 10 min).
2. Skim top of broth.
3. Add tomatoes, spinach and seasonings
4. Cook for 15 minutes on medium heat

This soup is one of my favorites. It is perfect for a nice hot lunch or dinner meal. I usually will make a large pot and freeze what I don't eat for another day.

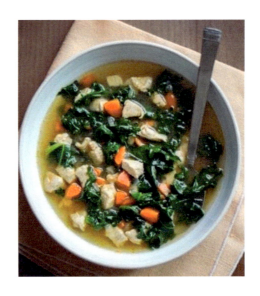

Desserts ☺

Note *** I will usually make a large batch of these and take with me in my lunch for a low to no carb treat ☺

Kimmie's Coconut-chocolate chip Cookies

4 oz cream cheese
2 eggs
1 tsp vanilla
1 tsp baking soda
1 c. Oat fiber
1 c. bitter sweet choc chips
1 c. toasted coconut
1 c. Truvia sweetener Preheat oven to 425.

1. Mix together all ingredients in mixer on medium speed until smooth.
2. Place in tablespoon spoons into a greased muffin pan
3. Bake for 14-18 min until golden brown.

- You can use coconut flour instead of the oat fiber however there will be added carbs.

Note* you can also add unsweetened cocoa powder to make these more chocolaty!! ☺

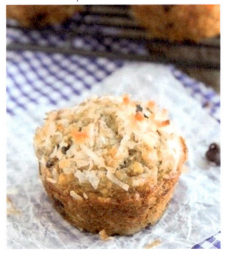

Salty Chocolate Treat

Here's a simple low-carb treat that is appreciated and easy to make for special occasions. 2 grams of carbs per serving

- 4 oz. 100 g dark chocolate with a minimum of 70% cocoa solids
- Pecan nuts or walnuts
- 2 tablespoons roasted unsweetened coconut chips Sea salt

1. Melt the chocolate in the microwave oven. Bring out 10 small cupcake liners, no bigger than 2 inches in diameter.
2. Add the chocolate to the cupcake liners.
3. Add nuts, coconut chips, seeds and lastly a few salt flakes if you like the saltier flavor.
4. Let cool and store in the refrigerator.

Tip!

If you don't have cupcake liners, you can just pour the chocolate in a small baking dish with parchment paper. Spread nuts and coconut flakes on top and when the chocolate has hardened, break up into nice uneven pieces. You can also add chili for flavor, and perhaps some dry berries like blueberries or goji berries.

"Ice Cream"

2 tbl spoons of Lite Cool Whip
1 c. your choice fruit
1 packet of Truvia sweetener (optional)

1. Mix all ingredients together and freeze for 1 hour

This sure is a life safer for me!!! I keep all my Cool whip in the freezer for a quick 'ice cream' treat. Even without the fruit it still takes like plain ice cream when frozen.

Note** I will also add unsweetened cocoa powder for chocolate ice cream or powdered peanut butter for an even special treat !!! ☺

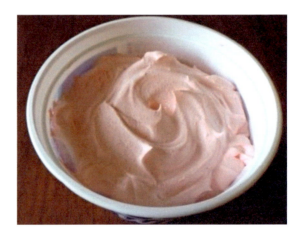

Orange Cranberry Muffins

3 eggs
4 oz of cream cheese
1 tsp baking powder
½ c Oat bran (optional)*
½ c dried cranberries
1 tsp vanilla
¼ c brown sugar (I use sukrin)

Preheat oven to 425

1. Combine all ingredients into a mixer and blend on high until smooth consistency
2. Spray muffin pan with cooking spray and fill ½ to top with muffin mixture
3. Bake for 18-20 min until golden brown

*Note: you can use almond flour or coconut flour, however there will be more carbs ☺

Dairy Free Coconut Cream w/Berries

½ cup Coconut cream
1 oz. 20 g fresh strawberries
1 pinch vanilla extract

With Raspberries
½ cup 1 dl coconut cream
1 oz. 20 g fresh raspberries
1 pinch vanilla extract

With Blueberries
½ cup 1 dl coconut cream
1½ oz. 50 g blueberries
1 pinch vanilla extract

Mix appropriate ingredients together, Enjoy ☺

Kimmie's Chocolate-frosted Cookies

2 ounces of cream cheese
1 ½ tsp vanilla
2 eggs
1 egg white
½ c. bittersweet chips
½ c. butter
2 tbls olive oil
¾ c. Truvia or ½ c sukrin sugar
1 ½ tsp Phyllum husk or 1 tsp xanthan gum
¼ c. cornstarch
½ c. oat fiber

Preheat oven to 375

1. Combine Oat fiber, corn starch & phyllum husk in a bowl. Set aside.
2. Combine sugar, cream cheese, butter & oil in a mixer & beat at medium speed until light and fluffy.
3. Add flour mixture, beat a t low speed until blended well.
4. Drop dough by spoonful 2 inches apart onto greased baking sheet. Bake at 375 for 13-15 minutes until cookies are lightly browned on edges.
5. Place chocolate chips in a microwave safe bowl for 1 min on high. Remove and stir. If needed microwave 15 more seconds until melted & smooth.
6. Spoon melted chocolate on each cookie and let set.

Note*…You can substitute coconut flour for Oat fiber, however carbs will be higher.

Low Carb Smoothies☺

Low Carb Smoothies
(ALL smoothies have 5 net carbs or less)

Strawberry Sage Smoothie

Blend 1 c of unsweetened coconut milk
5 frozen strawberries
2 tbsp heavy cream
1 fresh sage leaf (optional)
1 tsp sugar free vanilla syrup

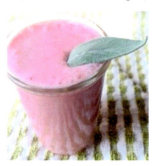

Cheesecake Smoothie

Blend 1 cup of almond milk
½ c raspberries
1 oz cream cheese
1 tblsp sugar free vanilla syrup

HAZELNUT COFFEE LATTE

Blend 1 cup cold coffee
½ c heavy cream
2 tbsp sugar free hazelnut syrup
Tons of ice cubes

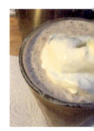

Salted Caramel Cashew Smoothie

Blend 1 Cup unsweetened cashew milk 3 tsp heavy cream 5 ice cubes 2 tbsp sugar free salted caramel syrup
Sprinkle with pumpkin pie spice

Strawberry Coconut Smoothie

Blend 1 cup unsweetened coconut milk
5 frozen strawberries
4 tbsp of heavy cream 2 tbsp sugar free vanilla syrup

Here are the pictures of the Sukrin syrup, Oat Fiber, and no carb pasta

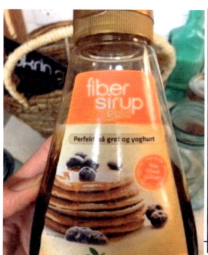
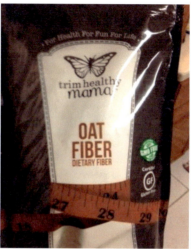
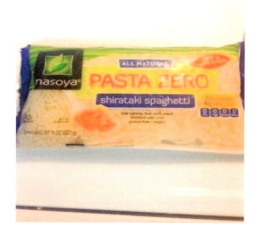

Note *** I buy the fiber sirup* and Oat Fiber on Amazon. The Pasta zero I buy at Publix and Walmart in the Tofu section near the fresh veggies.

Facts about Fiber Sirup: Sukrin Fiber Syrup Gold is a natural origin low calorie and low carb alternative to honey and syrup with the sweetness, flavor and taste of molasses/syrup. Sukrin Fiber Syrup Gold is suitable for: •Pancakes •Desserts• Yogurt •Ice Cream •In barbecue sauces •Coffee and tea• Made of a plant fiber called isomaltooligosaccharide (IMO), this syrup provides the very beneficial prebiotic fibres. A small amount of steviol glycosides is added to obtain the same sweetness as honey or sugar as well as a little bit of malt extract for color and fullness of taste •No artificial colors, additives or preservatives

Facts about Oat Fiber: This is a gluten-free, zero calorie flour full of dietary fiber. It is awesome to help save your yummy baked goodies from wreaking havoc on your waistline.

Facts about Pasta Zero: Shirataki noodles are known by many different names. They have sometimes been called "miracle noodles" because of two reasons: A Zero or Low Calorie Noodle. It is incredibly hard for many people to believe that there actually is a product in the noodle form that has either zero calories or absolutely no calories at all. If someone addicted to pasta or on a low cab diet is actively trying to lose weight, this can seem like a miracle product. The potential to eat just as much of this pasta as you would like without suffering a high calorie consequence have many people believing this is in an absolute miracle.

☺ Thank you for purchasing my book!!!! God Bless ☺

Made in the USA
Columbia, SC
07 June 2025